Overcoming Bronchiectasis

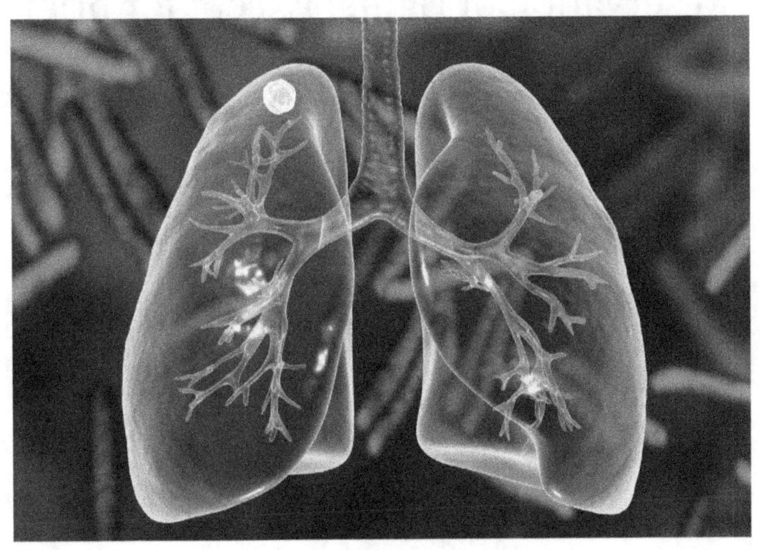

A Step-by-Step Guide to Beating Bronchiectasis for Patients and Health Care Providers

Rebecca J. Reynolds

Content

INTRODUCTION

Welcome to "Overcoming Bronchiectasis: A Step-by-Step Guide to Beating Bronchiectasis for Patients and Health Care Providers." This comprehensive guide is a beacon of empowerment for individuals facing the challenges of bronchiectasis, providing a roadmap to triumph over this respiratory condition.

Whether you are a patient navigating the complexities of bronchiectasis or a healthcare provider seeking insights and strategies, this book is designed to be your trusted companion. Together, we embark on a journey that demystifies bronchiectasis, offering a clear understanding of its nuances, treatment options, and proactive measures.

Bronchiectasis, a condition impacting the airways, demands a multidimensional approach to navigate its intricacies successfully. Throughout these pages, we will delve into the causes, symptoms, and diagnosis of bronchiectasis, equipping you with the knowledge needed to make informed decisions about your health.

Patients will find solace in practical advice on treatment options, preventive measures, and embracing a holistic mindset. Health care providers will discover valuable insights to enhance patient care, fostering a collaborative approach towards managing bronchiectasis effectively.

As we embark on this journey together, let "Overcoming Bronchiectasis" be your guide to resilience, empowerment, and triumph. Whether you are seeking self-help strategies or professional insights, this book is a testament to the strength that emerges when knowledge meets action. Let us navigate the path to overcoming bronchiectasis—one step at a time.

Purpose of the Book

The purpose of "Overcoming Bronchiectasis: A Step-by-Step Guide to Beating Bronchiectasis for Patients and Health Care Providers" is to serve as a comprehensive resource that empowers both patients and healthcare providers in their journey to conquer bronchiectasis. This book aims to:

1. Educate Patients: Provide a thorough understanding of bronchiectasis, its causes, symptoms, and the impact on respiratory health, enabling patients to make informed decisions about their well-being.

2. Empower with Practical Steps: Offer a step-by-step guide, equipping patients with actionable strategies to navigate their daily lives, manage symptoms, and actively participate in their treatment plans.

3.Facilitate Informed Collaboration:Foster a collaborative relationship between patients and healthcare providers by demystifying the diagnosis and treatment processes. The book encourages open communication and shared decision-making.

4. Guide Healthcare Providers: Equip healthcare professionals with insights into patient perspectives, facilitating more effective communication, personalized care, and improved patient outcomes.

5. Holistic Approach: Emphasize a holistic approach by incorporating not only medical interventions but also lifestyle adjustments, preventive measures, and natural remedies for a well-rounded and sustainable management of bronchiectasis.

In essence, this book serves as a beacon of knowledge, guidance, and empowerment for individuals navigating the challenges of bronchiectasis, fostering a proactive partnership between patients and healthcare providers on the path to overcoming this respiratory condition.

"Helen's Breath of Hope"

In a quaint town nestled between rolling hills and meandering streams, lived a woman named Helen. Helen had faced the challenges of bronchiectasis with unwavering determination and a spirit that refused to be dampened by the weight of her condition.

Helen's journey began with the diagnosis that changed her life. Yet, instead of letting it define her, she embraced the opportunity to learn and grow. Through the guidance of dedicated healthcare professionals, she discovered the beacon of hope called pulmonary rehabilitation.

In the heart of the town stood a warm and welcoming rehabilitation center, where Helen found not just exercise routines and medical advice, but a community of individuals sharing similar paths. She met others with bronchiectasis, forming bonds that transformed her perception of the condition from a burden to a shared challenge.

Under the guidance of compassionate healthcare providers, Helen engaged in tailored exercise programs, learning breathing techniques that felt like whispers of strength. The educational sessions illuminated the intricate details of bronchiectasis, empowering Helen with knowledge that became her shield against uncertainty.

Helen's journey wasn't without its hurdles. There were days when the weight of bronchiectasis felt heavier, but the camaraderie of her newfound community and the resilience she discovered within herself propelled her forward.

As weeks turned into months, Helen's transformation became evident. Her exercise tolerance improved, breathlessness became a memory, and the once-daunting coughs diminished. Pulmonary rehabilitation wasn't just about physical changes; it was a holistic metamorphosis that touched every facet of her being.

The ripple effect of Helen's journey extended beyond herself. She became a beacon of hope for others in her community, inspiring them to embark on their own paths of healing. With newfound vigor, she shared her story, demonstrating that bronchiectasis need not shroud life in darkness but could be a canvas for strength and resilience.

In this small town, Helen's breath of hope wafted through the air, touching the lives of those facing bronchiectasis. It was a testament to the power of community, education, and the indomitable human spirit that refuses to be defined by its challenges. Helen's story echoed through the hills, reminding everyone that, in the face of adversity, there is always a breath of hope waiting to be discovered.

How to phrase it

Brohng-kee-EHK-tuh-sihs

CHAPTER ONE

Understanding Bronchiectasis

What is bronchiectasis

Bronchiectasis is a condition that influences the aviation routes to the lungs. It's frequently brought about by scarring that came about because of a contamination or other fiery condition. You can be brought into the world with a condition that makes it bound to create. Bronchiectasis hurts the walls of the aviation routes. Over the long haul, they become scarred, excited, and augmented. They then, at that point, can't get out bodily fluid. This harm can prompt serious lung contaminations and other significant medical issues.

The aviation routes consist of a progression of spreading tubes. These are known as the bronchi, and the more modest ones are bronchioles. Through these cylinders, the lungs carry oxygen into the body. They likewise eliminate carbon dioxide from the body.

The aviation routes frequently have a covering of bodily fluid. This tacky substance assists with eliminating residue, microorganisms, and trash from the aviation routes. Small, hair-like designs (cilia) assist with moving the bodily fluid along. This cycle cleans up bodily fluid. After some time, you then gobble or hack it up.

Various circumstances, like contamination, can make bodily fluid development in the aviation routes. This development makes an optimal spot for microorganisms to develop. That can prompt more diseases. Each disease harms the aviation routes somewhat more. They are then bound to get another contamination.

After some time, these rehashed diseases can forever harm the walls of the aviation routes. The aviation routes are enlarged. They become scarred and thickened. Over the long run, they will be unable to move oxygen in the air from the lungs to the body. Anybody can create bronchiectasis. However, it is more normal in ladies. In youngsters, it influences more young men than young ladies.

What are the types of bronchiectasis

Bronchiectasis is classified into several types based on its underlying causes and associated conditions. Here are the main types:

Cylindrical Bronchiectasis:
Description: In this type, the airways become dilated, resembling the shape of a cylinder.
Causes: Often associated with recurring respiratory infections and inflammation.

Varicose Bronchiectasis:

Description: Characterized by irregular, dilated bronchi with alternating areas of constriction.
Causes: Typically linked to chronic infections, immune system dysfunction, or aspiration.

Cystic Bronchiectasis:
Description: Involves the formation of cyst-like spaces in the bronchial walls.
Causes: Commonly associated with genetic conditions such as cystic fibrosis.

Saccular Bronchiectasis:
Description: The bronchi form sac-like dilations, leading to weakened airway walls.
Causes: Often related to severe lung infections or obstructions.

Traction Bronchiectasis:
Description: Results from the pulling or stretching of the bronchi due to fibrosis in surrounding lung tissue.
Causes: Associated with conditions causing scarring of the lungs, like interstitial lung diseases.

Mucoid Impaction Bronchiectasis:

Description: Occurs when mucus becomes impacted within the bronchi, leading to dilation.
Causes: Typically seen in chronic conditions with excessive mucus production.

Post-infectious Bronchiectasis:

Description: Develops as a consequence of severe respiratory infections.
Causes: Previous infections, especially in childhood, can result in permanent bronchial damage.

Anatomy of the Respiratory System

The respiratory system is a complex network of organs and structures responsible for the exchange of oxygen and carbon dioxide, essential for sustaining life. Here is an overview of the anatomy of the respiratory system:

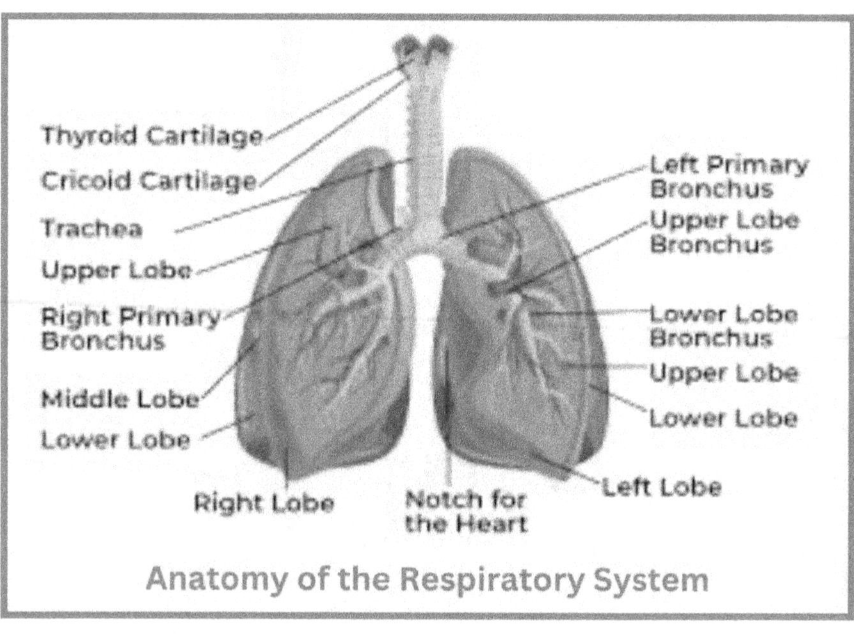

Anatomy of the Respiratory System

Nasal Cavity:
Function: Filters, humidifies, and warms incoming air.
Structures: Nostrils, nasal septum, turbinates.

Pharynx:
Function: Serves as a common pathway for both air and food.
Sections: Nasopharynx, oropharynx, laryngopharynx.

Larynx:
Function: Houses the vocal cords and ensures the separation of the airway and digestive tract.
Structures: Epiglottis, vocal cords.

Trachea:
Function: Conducts air from the larynx to the bronchi.
Structure: C-shaped cartilaginous rings for support.

Bronchial Tree:

Function: Divides into smaller airways, facilitating air distribution.

Structures: Primary bronchi, secondary bronchi, bronchioles.

Alveoli:

Function: Site of gas exchange (oxygen and carbon dioxide) with the bloodstream.

Structure: Tiny air sacs surrounded by capillaries.

Lungs:

Function: Main respiratory organs containing bronchial tree and alveoli.

Structures: Lobes (right lung has three lobes, left lung has two lobes).

Pleura:

Function: Membrane surrounding the lungs, reducing friction during breathing.

Structures: Visceral pleura (attached to the lungs), parietal pleura (lines the chest cavity).

Diaphragm:

Function: Primary muscle for breathing, contracting to increase lung volume during inhalation.
Structure: Dome-shaped muscle separating the chest and abdominal cavities.

Intercostal Muscles:
Function: Assist in expanding and contracting the chest during breathing.
Structures: Muscles between the ribs.

What's the difference between bronchiectasis and bronchitis

Bronchiectasis is a long-term condition characterized by the abnormal widening and damage to the bronchi, which are the airways leading to the lungs. This structural damage results in a reduced ability to clear mucus from the airways, leading to its accumulation. Persistent mucus build-up can become a breeding ground for bacteria, causing recurrent infections and inflammation.

On the contrary, bronchitis refers to the inflammation of the bronchial tubes, which are responsible for carrying air to the lungs. Bronchitis can be either acute or chronic. Acute bronchitis is often caused by viral infections, such as the common cold, while chronic bronchitis is typically associated with long-term exposure to irritants like smoking. Both types of bronchitis involve increased production of mucus, coughing, and difficulty breathing.

How your body is shielded by mucus

Mucus serves as a crucial protective barrier in your body. Produced by goblet cells in various mucous membranes, such as those in the respiratory and digestive systems, mucus plays a multifaceted role in shielding your body.

In the respiratory system, for instance, mucus acts as a first line of defense by trapping inhaled particles, microbes, and irritants. Cilia, tiny hair-like structures, then move in coordinated waves to propel the mucus and its trapped cargo away from the airways. This mechanism helps prevent foreign substances from reaching deeper into the lungs, reducing the risk of infections and maintaining respiratory health.

Moreover, in the digestive tract, mucus lubricates and protects the lining of the stomach and intestines. It helps in the smooth passage of food, preventing irritation and damage to the delicate tissues. Additionally, mucus contains enzymes and antibodies that contribute to the body's immune defense, neutralizing potential threats.

In essence, the production of mucus serves as a dynamic defense mechanism, aiding in the prevention of infections, supporting the function of various organs, and contributing to the overall well-being of the body.

CHAPTER TWO

Causes and Triggers

Imagine your lungs like an intricate network of branching tubes carrying air to your lungs, like tiny highways for oxygen. These tubes are called bronchi. In bronchiectasis, these highways get damaged and widen, becoming like misshapen, bumpy roads. This makes it harder for your lungs to clear mucus and germs, leading to infections, coughing, and other problems.

There are several ways these "highways" can get damaged, like:

Infections: Think of a bad case of pneumonia that scars the inside of your bronchi. These scars can cause them to widen and become less efficient.

Immune system issues: Sometimes, your body's defense system isn't strong enough to fight off infections, making your bronchi more vulnerable to damage.

Genetic conditions: Some people are born with conditions that affect the cilia, tiny hairs inside the bronchi that help move mucus. Without proper cilia, mucus gets stuck, leading to inflammation and eventually widening.

Other factors: Inhaling harmful substances like dust or chemicals, or suffering from certain lung diseases like cystic fibrosis, can also damage the bronchi.

Once damaged, the widened bronchi trap mucus and germs, making you more prone to infections. This cycle of infections and further damage can lead to various symptoms like:

- Chronic cough with thick mucus
- Wheezing
- Shortness of breath
- Chest pain
- Fatigue

Okay, let's put on our detective hats and dig deeper into the genetic clues of bronchiectasis!

Genetic Factors

Imagine your genes like a blueprint for building your body. Sometimes, there can be tiny typos or missing lines in that blueprint, and one such typo can affect the cilia in your lungs. These little guys are like tiny hair brushes lining your airways, constantly sweeping away mucus and germs. If they don't work properly due to the typo in your genes, mucus gets stuck, leading to infections and eventually those widened, bumpy "highways" we talked about earlier.

This genetic typo can be inherited from your parents, just like the color of your eyes or hair. But don't worry, even with this typo, not everyone gets bronchiectasis. Think of it like adding a bit of spice to your genetic stew - it might add some flavor, but it doesn't necessarily mean the whole pot will be spicy!

Genetic factors play a role in bronchiectasis, a condition characterized by permanent enlargement of the airways. Mutations in genes related to the immune system, cilia function, or connective tissue integrity can contribute to the development of bronchiectasis. These genetic abnormalities may impair the respiratory system's ability to defend against infections, leading to recurrent lung infections and eventual bronchiectasis. Additionally, individuals with a family history of bronchiectasis are at a higher risk due to shared genetic susceptibility.

Environmental Influences

Imagine your lungs like a beautiful garden full of healthy plants (the bronchi). These plants work hard to keep the garden free of weeds and pests (mucus and germs). But sometimes, harsh winds (environmental factors) can damage the delicate branches and leaves of the plants. This makes it harder for them to keep the garden clean, leading to weeds and pests thriving, just like infections and breathing problems in bronchiectasis.

Here are some ways the "harsh winds" of the environment can harm your lung garden:

Toxic Air: Breathing in dust, chemicals, or pollution can irritate and inflame the bronchi, making them weak and vulnerable to infections. Imagine breathing in smoke from a bonfire – that's how harsh these airborne irritants can be!

Secondhand Smoke: Like a lingering wildfire, secondhand smoke damages the delicate lining of the bronchi, increasing the risk of infections and bronchiectasis.

Occupational Exposures: Some jobs involve working with harmful substances like asbestos or silica dust. These can be like mini-tornadoes in your lungs, causing significant damage to the bronchi over time.

Poor Air Quality: Living in areas with high levels of air pollution can be like constantly walking through a dusty desert for your lungs. This constant exposure to irritants can wear down the bronchi and make them more susceptible to infections.

It's important to remember that environmental factors often work together with other causes of bronchiectasis, like infections or genetic conditions. Think of it like a storm hitting a weakened tree – both the internal weakness and the external force contribute to the damage.

Note: While infections and genetics play a role, environmental factors like pollution, smoke, and occupational exposures can significantly contribute to bronchiectasis. Taking steps to avoid these "harsh winds" by wearing masks, choosing cleaner environments, and advocating for air quality improvements can help protect your lung garden and keep it healthy.

CHAPTER TWO

Recognizing Symptoms

Remember your lung garden from before? When something goes wrong, the plants send out signals to let you know they're in trouble. In bronchiectasis, your lungs do the same, sending out symptoms like:

The Chronic Cough:

Imagine a gardener constantly clearing their throat as leaves and twigs clog the paths. That's what the chronic cough of bronchiectasis feels like. It's usually productive, meaning it brings up mucus, which can be yellow, green, or even foul-smelling.

Wheezing like a Rusty Gate:

Remember that old creaky gate in the garden? Wheezing sounds like that, a whistling or rattling noise when you breathe. It happens because the widened bronchi make it harder for air to flow freely.

Shortness of Breath:

Think of taking a long hike uphill with heavy bags. That's how shortness of breath in bronchiectasis feels. It's because damaged bronchi limit the amount of oxygen that reaches your body, making even simple activities feel tiring.

Feeling Fatigued:

Imagine working all day in the garden without enough sunlight. That's how fatigue feels in bronchiectasis. Your body is constantly fighting infections and clearing mucus, draining your energy.

Chest Pain:

Think of pulling a weed and feeling a little tug.
Chest pain in bronchiectasis feels like that, a dull
ache or sharp pain caused by inflammation or
muscle strain from coughing.

Other Clues:

Sometimes, the garden sends subtler signals. Look
for frequent chest infections, unexplained weight
loss, clubbing of the fingertips (where the nail beds
become rounded), or even nosebleeds.

Chronic Cough

Imagine tending your beautiful lung garden, filled
with delicate plants representing your airways.
Suddenly, a persistent cough erupts, like a
relentless wind rattling the leaves and disrupting
the peaceful harmony. This, unfortunately, is the
hallmark of bronchiectasis – a chronic cough that
simply won't quit.

Unlike the occasional cough we all experience, this insistent gardener's cough has distinct features:

- A stubborn resident: This cough sticks around for weeks, months, or even years,refusing to take a vacation.
- The phlegm parade: It's rarely solo, often accompanied by a parade of mucus,ranging from clear to yellow, green, or even foul-smelling, hinting at trouble in the garden.
- More than just a clearing: This cough isn't a gentle breeze but a forceful gust,sometimes causing chest pain or even exhaustion.
- A disruptive guest: It disrupts sleep,interferes with daily activities, and can affect your social life, making you feel like a gardener constantly weeding a neglected patch.

But why this relentless cough? Remember the widened, damaged bronchi from our previous analogy? They become like tangled pathways, trapping mucus and germs, triggering the cough reflex to try and clear the clutter. This cycle of

infection and inflammation keeps the cough going,
making it your unwelcome, persistent guest.

Here's the key:

- Don't ignore the gardener: A chronic cough,
  especially with mucus, shouldn't be
  dismissed as a simple cold. See a doctor.
- Early diagnosis matters: Identifying
  bronchiectasis early allows for timely
  treatment, helping to control the
  cough,prevent complications, and improve
  your quality of life.
- Treat the cause, not just the
  cough:Medications help manage infections
  and inflammation, but addressing the
  underlying cause, like environmental factors
  or genetic conditions, is crucial for
  long-term relief.

Remember, a healthy lung garden thrives on care
and attention. If your cough becomes the
persistent gardener, listen to its message. Seek
help, get diagnosed, and work with your doctor to

restore calm and peace to your inner garden. Your lungs, and your overall health, will thank you for it.

Excessive Sputum Production

Excessive sputum production is a common symptom of bronchiectasis, which means the airways in the lungs are permanently widened. In simpler terms, it leads to more mucus being made. Think of sputum as thick, sticky goo produced by the lungs. When someone has bronchiectasis, their airways make too much of this goo, making it harder for them to breathe. This excess mucus can also lead to frequent coughing and a feeling of chest congestion, making it an important sign to watch for if someone suspects they might have bronchiectasis.

Shortness of Breath

Imagine running through a dense forest, branches whipping past your face, your lungs burning for air. That's what shortness of breath in bronchiectasis can feel like – a constant struggle to fill your lungs, a desperate yearning for a normal breath.

This air hunger, known as dyspnea, is one of the most common and distressing symptoms of bronchiectasis. Unlike the occasional puff you might need after climbing stairs, this breathlessness lingers, intruding on every activity, from walking to talking.

But why does this happen? Picture your lungs as a network of delicate pathways, the bronchi. In bronchiectasis, these pathways are damaged and widen, becoming like distorted tunnels. This makes it harder for air to flow freely, like trying to breathe through a clogged straw.

Here's how this translates to breathlessness:

- Less Air Reaching Your Lungs: **The wider,scarred bronchi offer less surface area for oxygen absorption. It's like having fewer leaves in your lung garden to capture sunlight (oxygen).**
- Mucus Blockage: **The damaged bronchi trap mucus more easily, creating further hurdles for air to navigate. Imagine twigs and debris blocking the paths in your garden.**
- Inflammation: **The constant battle against infections and mucus irritates and inflames the bronchi, causing them to tighten and further restrict airflow. Think of thorns pricking the delicate branches of your lung plants.**

This struggle for air can manifest in different ways:

- Constant feeling of not getting enough air, even while resting
- Difficulty catching your breath, especially after exertion
- Rapid, shallow breathing
- Tightness or pressure in your chest
- Wheezing, a whistling or rattling sound when you breathe

Remember, shortness of breath in bronchiectasis is not just about feeling winded. It's a sign that your lungs are struggling, and it's crucial to seek medical attention. Early diagnosis and treatment can help manage the condition, reduce inflammation, and make breathing easier, allowing you to reclaim your breath and enjoy life without constant air hunger.

What diseases cause bronchiectasis

Imagine your lungs as a bustling city, with airways like busy streets carrying vital oxygen throughout. In bronchiectasis, these highways become damaged and widen, causing congestion and chaos. But who are the culprits behind this lung-city mayhem? Let's meet the common suspects:

The Infection Gang:

Pneumonia: This lung infection can leave scars that weaken the airways, paving the way for bronchiectasis. Think of it like a pothole left unrepaired, disrupting traffic flow.

Pertussis (Whooping Cough): This highly contagious bacterial infection inflames and damages the airways, making them vulnerable to widening and mucus build-up. It's like a traffic jam caused by reckless drivers!

Tuberculosis (TB): This chronic bacterial infection can scar and destroy lung tissue,including the airways, leading to bronchiectasis. Imagine buildings collapsing and blocking crucial routes.

The Immune System Squad:

Cystic Fibrosis: This genetic condition affects how mucus moves in the airways,causing it to become thick and sticky,leading to infections and airway damage.Picture traffic clogged by molasses-like sludge.

Immunodeficiency Disorders: Conditions like HIV or hypogammaglobulinemia weaken your immune system, making you more susceptible to lung infections that can damage the airways, like rogue vehicles causing accidents.

The Inherited Trait Crew:

Primary Ciliary Dyskinesia (PCD): This genetic condition affects the tiny hairs (cilia) in the airways that help clear mucus.Without proper ciliary movement, mucus stagnates, causing inflammation and airway widening. Think of malfunctioning street sweepers leaving debris to pile up.

The Environmental Enforcers:

Exposure to Harmful Substances: Chronic inhalation of dust, chemicals, or pollution can irritate and damage the airways, increasing the risk of bronchiectasis. Imagine smog choking the city streets.

Note:

Often, bronchiectasis is caused by a combination of these factors, not just one. Think of a perfect storm brewing from various sources.

CHAPTER Three

Diagnosis and Tests

Imagine your lungs as a vibrant marketplace bustling with activity, air flowing freely through delicate pathways like bustling streets. In bronchiectasis, these pathways become damaged and widen, causing congestion and disruption. But how do we identify this hidden disarray? Let's dive into the fascinating world of diagnosis, unearthing the methods used to pinpoint and understand bronchiectasis.

Imaging Techniques

Bronchiectasis is a lung condition where the airways become abnormally widened and damaged, making it difficult to clear mucus and fight off infections. Imagine your bronchial tubes, the "highways" in your lungs, being stretched and scarred, leading to traffic jams of sticky mucus.

Diagnosing bronchiectasis relies heavily on imaging techniques that allow doctors to take a peek inside your lungs and see what's going on.

Here are the main players in the imaging game for bronchiectasis:

1. Chest X-ray: This classic black and white image is like a quick snapshot of your lungs. While not the best detective for bronchiectasis, it can be a helpful first step, sometimes showing signs like thickened bronchial walls or air trapping.

2. High-resolution Computed Tomography (HRCT): Think of HRCT as a super-powered X-ray. It uses radiation to create detailed cross-sectional images of your lungs, much like thin slices of bread revealing the inner crumb. This is the gold standard for diagnosing bronchiectasis, as it can clearly show the dilated, irregular airways and other telltale signs like mucus plugs.

3. Bronchoscopy: This technique involves inserting a thin, flexible tube with a camera (bronchoscope) through your mouth or nose and down into your airways. It's like sending a tiny explorer to map the bronchial "tunnels" directly. While not commonly used for diagnosis, bronchoscopy can be helpful in some cases to see blockages or take tissue samples.

4. Nuclear Medicine Scans: These specialized scans use radioactive tracers to assess lung function and blood flow. They can be helpful in identifying underlying causes of bronchiectasis, such as inflammation or scarring.

Choosing the right imaging technique depends on various factors:

- Your symptoms and medical history
- The doctor's suspicion of bronchiectasis

- Available resources and expertise

Remember, these imaging tools are just pieces of the puzzle. A doctor's expertise in interpreting the images and correlating them with your clinical picture is crucial for an accurate diagnosis of bronchiectasis.

Beyond diagnosis, imaging also plays a vital role in:

- Assessing the severity of bronchiectasis
- Identifying underlying causes
- Monitoring disease progression and treatment response

So, the next time you suspect something might be wrong with your lungs, remember that these imaging techniques can be your allies in uncovering the mysteries within. They may not be as thrilling as X-ray vision from comic books, but they offer a powerful glimpse into your lung health, paving the way for proper diagnosis and treatment of bronchiectasis.

Pulmonary Function Tests

Imagine your lungs as giant balloons constantly filling and emptying with air. In bronchiectasis, these balloons get wonky. The tubes (bronchi) leading to the balloons (air sacs) become damaged and stretched, like balloons with weak necks. This makes it hard for air to get all the way in and out, causing coughing, breathlessness, and other nasty symptoms.

Pulmonary function tests (PFTs) are like special tools that doctors use to peek inside your lung balloons and see how well they're doing. These tests are like blowing party horns, but instead of confetti, they measure how much air you can blow and how fast you can do it.

Here's how different PFTs help diagnose bronchiectasis:

1. Spirometry: This is the star of the show! You blow into a mouthpiece while wearing nose clips (think fancy laundry pegs), like blowing out birthday candles on a giant cake. The spirometer measures how much air you can blow out in one second (FEV1) and how much you can blow out in total

(FVC). In bronchiectasis, your FEV1 might be lower than the FVC, making the "cake" lopsided.

2. Plethysmography: This test goes beyond blowing. You sit in a special box and wear a snug bodysuit that measures your chest and belly movements as you breathe. It's like having a hug from a measuring tape! This helps assess how much air your lungs can hold and how well they inflate with each breath.

3. Diffusion Capacity: This one checks how good your lungs are at transferring oxygen from the air you breathe into your blood. Imagine tiny mailboxes delivering oxygen packages from the air to your red blood cell postman. In bronchiectasis, these mailboxes might be damaged, slowing down the delivery of oxygen packages.

4. X-ray and CT Scan: These are like powerful flashlights shining through your chest, helping doctors see if your lung balloons are misshapen or if there's any mucus plugging them up.

Putting it all together: PFTs give doctors a snapshot of how your lungs are working. In bronchiectasis, the spirometry results are often the most telling. But, like clues in a detective story, doctors consider all the PFTs and scans together to make a diagnosis.

 Note: PFTs can't cure bronchiectasis, but they're crucial tools for monitoring your condition and guiding treatment. They help doctors see if your lung balloons are getting stronger or weaker and adjust your treatment accordingly.

 So, the next time you hear about PFTs, don't be scared! Think of them as your allies in the fight against bronchiectasis, helping you breathe easier and live a fuller life.

Consultation with Healthcare Professionals

Bronchiectasis, a lung condition where airways become abnormally widened and damaged, can be tricky to diagnose. But fear not, consulting a healthcare professional plays a crucial role in

unraveling this mystery and leading you towards
the right path. Think of it as a detective story, where
the healthcare professional is the master sleuth,
using various clues to pinpoint the culprit –
bronchiectasis.

The Initial Interview:

Your first consultation will be like laying the
groundwork for the investigation. The healthcare
professional will ask detailed questions about your
symptoms, like:

Persistent cough: Is it productive (with mucus) or
dry? How long have you had it?

Sputum: Mucus coughed up – its color, amount,
and any foul odor.

Chest pain or discomfort.

Breathing difficulties: Shortness of breath,
wheezing, or difficulty clearing mucus.
Fever, weight loss, or fatigue.

These questions help paint a picture of your overall
health and provide early clues.

Next, the detective (healthcare professional) gathers more evidence through various tests:

Physical examination: Listening to your lungs with a stethoscope to detect abnormal sounds like crackles or wheezes.
Chest X-ray: An initial snapshot of your lungs, revealing any airway widening or scarring.
Sputum test: Analyzing the mucus coughed up to identify any infections or bacteria.
Lung function tests: Measuring how well your lungs are working and detecting airflow limitations.

High-resolution computed tomography (HRCT scan):
A detailed 3D image of your lungs, particularly helpful in diagnosing bronchiectasis.
These tests act as magnifying glasses, allowing the healthcare professional to delve deeper and gather concrete evidence.

Putting the Pieces Together:

Once all the clues are gathered, the healthcare professional analyzes them like a seasoned detective. They consider your symptoms, test results, and medical history to build a logical picture. Some key pieces of evidence for bronchiectasis include:

- Chronic cough with productive sputum.
- Widened and damaged airways seen on HRCT scan.
- Recurring chest infections.

- Airflow limitations on lung function tests.

By carefully examining all these pieces, the healthcare professional arrives at a diagnosis, confirming or ruling out bronchiectasis.

Your healthcare provider may do several tests to diagnose bronchiectasis or rule out other conditions, including:

CT or chest x-ray: Your healthcare provider will use a machine to take pictures of your lungs to determine if your airways are damaged. Blood test and sputum culture. Your healthcare provider will

take a sample of blood or mucus (sputum) to check
for infection. Pulmonary function tests. Your
provider will use lung function tests to determine
how well your lungs are working. Breathe into a
machine that measures your lung function.

DNA test: Your healthcare provider may take
a sample of blood or other body fluids to test for a
disease.

Sweat chloride test: If your doctor
thinks you may have cystic fibrosis, he or she will
do a sweat test. Sweat your hands or feet and take
a sample to check for signs of cystic fibrosis.
Bronchoscopy. In some cases, healthcare
professionals may use a procedure to take a closer
look at the airways (bronchoscopy). They use a
bronchoscope (a long, flexible tube with a light and
a camera at the end) to take samples of mucus or
pus from the lungs and examine them for anything
blocking the airways.

CHAPTER FOUR

Treatment Options

How is bronchiectasis treated

Bronchiectasis can't be totally restored, yet the side effects can be dealt with. Medical services suppliers treat bronchiectasis by eliminating bodily fluid and controlling contamination. Contingent upon the seriousness of the condition, your PCP might recommend prescription or non-intrusive treatment. You can likewise utilize clinical items to assist with eliminating the bodily fluid. Assuming bronchiectasis is brought about by a basic condition, treating that condition might help your side effects. In the event that the area of bronchiectasis is little, your PCP might suggest a medical procedure, yet this is uncommon.

Medications Overview

Medicine is often used to treat bronchiectasis. You may likewise require non-intrusive treatment. You ought to remain hydrated, as well. Keeping the mucus from thickening, which can make it difficult to cough up, can be helped by drinking enough water.

A few potential drugs you might take are:

Physiotherapy
Postural drainage and chest percussion therapy
can help loosen and clear mucus. Breathing
exercises help open the airways.

Medical equipment.
Oscillating expiratory pressure (PEP) devices and
shock vests break down and clear mucus from the
lungs.

Antibiotics:
Antibiotics are used to treat bacterial illnesses.
medicines can be taken as pills, but if you have a
serious illness, your doctor will inject medicines
straight into your bloodstream via an IV. In addition,
doctors frequently recommend inhaled antibiotics to
treat bronchiectasis. For inhaled drugs, you can use
a nebulizer to turn the medication into a mist that
you breathe in.

Breathed in steroids.
These reduce inflammation (often combined with
bronchodilators in the same inhaler).

Expectorants and bodily fluid thinners:
These assist with slackening the bodily fluid in the
lungs and make it simpler to hack up.

These assist with facilitating blockage.

Chest active recuperation is one more significant piece of treatment. It incorporates beating your chest and back over and over to release the bodily fluid from your lungs. You may likewise learn exceptional breathing techniques. These can move the bodily fluid into the upper piece of your aviation route so you can hack it up. Your medical services supplier may likewise prompt utilizing a handheld or wearable gadget. These assistance move and clear bodily fluid from your lungs. There are many devices available. Your supplier will let you know the choices that are best for you.

Oxygen therapy may be needed by some people. Oxygen levels in their blood might be excessively low. Surgery may also be recommended by your healthcare provider. It might very well be a choice in the event that different medicines haven't worked and the condition is disengaged in one region of the lung. In uncommon cases, you could require a lung relocation.

The severity of your symptoms, your other health conditions, and other factors will all play a role in your treatment plan. Early finding and treatment can prevent the condition from deteriorating.

Pulmonary Rehabilitation

Pulmonary rehabilitation, often abbreviated as "pulm rehab," plays a vital role in managing bronchiectasis, a chronic lung condition marked by dilated airways and recurrent infections. While there's no cure for bronchiectasis, pulm rehab offers a powerful set of tools to improve symptoms, quality of life, and overall lung health.

What is Pulmonary Rehabilitation

Pulm rehab is a comprehensive program designed to help individuals with chronic lung conditions like bronchiectasis manage their symptoms and live fuller lives. It typically involves a combination of:

Exercise training: Tailored exercises to improve exercise tolerance, muscle strength, and endurance. This may include walking, cycling, swimming, or other activities the individual enjoys.

Education: Workshops and sessions provide knowledge about bronchiectasis, managing symptoms, coping strategies, and healthy lifestyle habits.

Psychological support: Individual or group therapy sessions can address anxiety, depression, and other emotional challenges associated with chronic illness.

Nutritional counseling: Proper nutrition is crucial for maintaining lung health and managing flare-ups. A dietician can provide personalized guidance.

Disease management training: Learning self-management techniques like airway clearance exercises, medication management, and identifying early signs of flare-ups.

Benefits of Pulmonary Rehabilitation for Bronchiectasis:

Improved exercise capacity: Pulm rehab helps individuals with bronchiectasis exercise for longer periods and with greater ease, reducing breathlessness and fatigue.

Reduced symptom burden: The program can alleviate symptoms like cough, wheezing, and sputum production, leading to a better quality of life.
Enhanced emotional well-being: Education and support can lessen anxiety and depression, boosting overall well-being and coping skills.

Decreased hospitalization rates: Studies show that pulm rehab reduces the need for hospital admissions due to bronchiectasis flare-ups.

Increased independence and participation in daily activities: Improved stamina and symptom control allow individuals to regain independence and engage in activities they enjoy.
Who is eligible for Pulmonary Rehabilitation?

Pulm rehab is beneficial for most individuals with bronchiectasis, regardless of the severity of their condition. It's particularly helpful for those who:

- Experience significant limitations in daily activities due to breathlessness or fatigue.
- Have frequent exacerbations or hospital admissions.
- Struggle with emotional challenges like anxiety or depression related to their condition.
- Are motivated to improve their health and well-being.

What to Expect During Pulmonary Rehabilitation:

Pulm rehab programs typically last for 6-12 weeks, with sessions held 2-3 times per week. The program is individualized to cater to each person's specific needs and abilities. It can be conducted in various settings, including hospitals, outpatient clinics, or even community centers.

Making the Most of Pulmonary Rehabilitation:

Active participation: Regular attendance and active participation in all aspects of the program are crucial for optimal results.

Open communication: Communicate openly with your healthcare team about your progress, any challenges you face, and any questions you may have.

Maintaining exercise after completion: Continue incorporating the learned exercises into your daily routine to sustain the benefits of the program. Lifestyle changes: Implement the dietary and lifestyle recommendations provided to support overall lung health and well-being.

Pulmonary rehabilitation is a valuable and effective treatment option for individuals with bronchiectasis. It empowers them to manage their symptoms, improve their quality of life, and breathe easier with every step. If you are living with bronchiectasis, talk to your doctor about whether pulm rehab is right for you.

Surgical Interventions

While not a first-line treatment for bronchiectasis, surgery can offer significant benefits for certain patients with severe, localized disease that hasn't responded to optimal medical management. Here's a comprehensive overview of surgical options for bronchiectasis:

Indications for Surgery:

Localized bronchiectasis: When only a specific part of the lung is affected, surgery to remove that portion can significantly improve symptoms and prevent future infections.

Severe symptoms: Chronic cough, hemoptysis (coughing up blood), recurrent lung infections, and significant decline in lung function despite maximal medical therapy could benefit from surgery.

Complications: Uncontrolled bleeding, pneumothorax (collapsed lung), or emphysema are potential indications for surgery.

Types of Surgical Procedures:

Lobectomy: Removal of an entire lobe of the lung is the most common surgery for bronchiectasis. Segmentectomy: Removal of a smaller section of a lung lobe is preferred when possible, minimizing lung tissue loss.

Pneumonectomy: Removal of an entire lung is rarely performed and only in highly complex cases.

Lung volume reduction surgery (LVRS): For emphysema cases associated with bronchiectasis, this procedure removes damaged lung tissue to improve breathing.

Minimally Invasive Approaches:

Video-assisted thoracoscopic surgery (VATS): Using small incisions and a camera, VATS offers faster recovery, less pain, and shorter hospital stays compared to traditional open surgery.

Robotic-assisted thoracic surgery: Similar to VATS, but robots assist the surgeon, potentially leading to greater precision and shorter operative times.

Outcomes and Considerations:

Success rates: Surgical outcomes are generally good, with significant symptom improvement and reduced infection rates in appropriately selected patients.

Risks and complications: Like any surgery, there are potential risks of bleeding, infection, pain, and respiratory complications.

Preoperative evaluation: Extensive testing and careful consideration are crucial to determine if surgery is suitable and ensure optimal success.

Postoperative care: Rehabilitation and supportive therapy are essential for complete recovery and long-term lung health.

Remember: Surgery is not a cure for bronchiectasis, and patients will still need ongoing medical management to prevent new infections and manage remaining lung function.

CHAPTER SIX

Preventive Measures

Bronchiectasis, a chronic lung condition marked by dilated airways, while not completely preventable, can be significantly influenced by proactive measures you take throughout your life. Here's a comprehensive guide to preventive measures for bronchiectasis:

Early Intervention:

Prompt diagnosis and treatment of underlying conditions:
Identifying and addressing factors like cystic fibrosis, autoimmune diseases, or recurrent lung infections early can prevent or slow the progression of bronchiectasis.

Childhood immunizations: Ensure you and your children are up-to-date on vaccinations for measles, whooping cough, and pneumococcal infections, which can contribute to bronchiectasis development.

Avoidance of harmful substances: Steer clear of smoke from cigarettes, vaping, and air pollution, as these irritate and damage the airways.

Healthy living: Maintain a balanced diet rich in fruits, vegetables, and whole grains while limiting processed foods and sugary drinks. Regular physical activity strengthens the respiratory system and overall health.

Good hygiene: Regular hand washing and maintaining distance from individuals with respiratory infections can prevent the spread of harmful bacteria and viruses.

Managing other health conditions: Address allergies, sinus infections, and other respiratory issues promptly to prevent them from contributing to bronchiectasis progression.

Lung Health Maintenance:

Mucus clearance techniques: Learn and practice techniques like chest physiotherapy, postural drainage, and percussion therapy to clear excess mucus from your airways, preventing buildup and infection.

Hydration: Drink plenty of fluids throughout the day to thin mucus and make it easier to cough up.

Pulmonary rehabilitation: This program, led by healthcare professionals, offers education, exercise training, and support to manage symptoms, improve lung function, and maintain quality of life.

Proactive Monitoring:

Regular follow-up with your doctor: Schedule regular checkups to monitor lung function, symptoms, and potential complications.
Early recognition of flare-ups: Be aware of signs like increased cough, sputum production, wheezing, and fever, and promptly seek medical attention to prevent worsening of symptoms.

Additional Considerations:

Occupational hazards: If your work exposes you to dust, fumes, or chemicals, wearing protective gear and ensuring proper ventilation are crucial.

Mental health and stress management: Chronic conditions like bronchiectasis can affect mental well-being. Practices like stress management techniques and seeking support groups can improve overall health and quality of life.

Note: While bronchiectasis is a chronic condition, proactive preventive measures can significantly improve your well-being and slow its progression. By adopting healthy lifestyle practices, avoiding harmful exposures, and managing your lung health, you can take control and live a fulfilling life.

Lifestyle Adjustments

Here are essential lifestyle adjustments that can play a significant role in preventive measures:

1. Smoking Cessation:

Smoking irritates the airways, worsens mucus production, and significantly accelerates bronchiectasis progression. Quitting smoking is the single most impactful preventive measure. Seek support groups, medications, or therapy to achieve smoking cessation.

2. Vaccination:

Regular flu and pneumococcal vaccinations are crucial. These vaccines offer protection against common respiratory infections that can trigger bronchiectasis flare-ups and worsen symptoms. Consult your doctor about recommended vaccination schedules.

3. Hygiene and Infection Control:

Frequent handwashing, especially after contact with sick individuals or public surfaces, reduces the risk of contracting respiratory infections.
Maintain good home hygiene by regularly cleaning surfaces, disinfecting frequently used items, and airing out your living space to minimize dust and allergen exposure.
Avoid close contact with individuals exhibiting signs of respiratory illness and crowded spaces during flu season.

4. Air Quality Management:

Avoid exposure to air pollutants like smog, smoke, and dust, which can irritate the airways and trigger flare-ups. Use air purifiers indoors, wear masks when air quality is poor, and avoid exposure to allergens like pollen and mold spores.

5. Nutrition and Hydration:

Maintain a healthy diet rich in fruits, vegetables, and whole grains to boost your immune system and overall health.
Stay hydrated by drinking plenty of water throughout the day. Adequate hydration thins mucus, making it easier to clear and reducing infection risk.

6. Regular Exercise:

Engaging in regular physical activity, like walking, swimming, or gentle yoga, can improve lung function, loosen mucus, and boost overall well-being. Consult your doctor about a safe and suitable exercise program for your individual needs.

7. Managing Underlying Conditions:

Address any underlying conditions like cystic fibrosis, allergies, or sinus infections that contribute to bronchiectasis. Effectively managing these conditions can indirectly prevent bronchiectasis flare-ups and progression.

8. Stress Management:

Chronic stress can weaken the immune system and exacerbate bronchiectasis symptoms. Learn stress-management techniques like meditation, yoga, or deep breathing exercises to promote relaxation and emotional well-being.

9. Regular Follow-up with your Doctor:

Scheduling regular check-ups with your doctor allows for monitoring lung function, symptom progression, and early identification of potential infections. Be proactive in communicating any changes you experience and adhere to prescribed medications and treatment plans.

10. Pulmonary Rehabilitation:

Consider participating in a pulmonary rehabilitation program if recommended by your doctor. This program offers supervised exercise training, education, and support to help manage symptoms, improve lung function, and enhance quality of life.

Remember, consistency and proactive effort are key to success in bronchiectasis prevention. By incorporating these lifestyle adjustments into your daily routine, you can significantly reduce the risk of flare-ups, infections, and disease progression, enabling you to live a fuller life with bronchiectasis.

Immunizations and Boosting Immunity

Immunizations and boosting overall immunity play a crucial role in this preventive approach.

Importance of Immunizations:

Reducing Infection Risk: Bronchiectasis patients are highly susceptible to respiratory infections, which can exacerbate symptoms and damage lung function. Regular vaccinations are vital to minimize this risk.

Specific Targets:

Influenza Vaccines: Annual flu shots are crucial, as influenza can trigger severe flare-ups in bronchiectasis patients.

Pneumococcal Vaccines: Vaccination against pneumococcal bacteria, another major cause of lung infections, is highly recommended.

Other Vaccines: Depending on individual risk factors and regional prevalence, additional vaccinations like measles, mumps, rubella, and whooping cough might be advisable.

Boosting General Immunity:

Healthy Lifestyle:

Balanced Diet: Prioritize fruits, vegetables, and whole grains for essential nutrients to support immune function.

Regular Exercise: Moderate physical activity helps boost circulation and enhances immune response.

Quality Sleep: Adequate sleep is crucial for immune system repair and regeneration.

Stress Management: Chronic stress can impair immune function. Relaxation techniques like yoga or meditation can help manage stress and enhance overall well-being.

Smoking Cessation: Smoking significantly weakens the respiratory system and worsens bronchiectasis. Quitting is essential for lung health and a strong immune system.

Hygiene Practices: Frequent handwashing and avoiding close contact with sick individuals can significantly reduce the risk of respiratory infections.

Environmental Considerations

Managing environmental triggers can play a crucial role in preventing infections, reducing symptom severity, and slowing disease progression. Here's a comprehensive overview of key environmental considerations and preventive measures:

Air Quality:

- **Minimize exposure to air pollutants:**
    - Avoid smoking and secondhand smoke.
    - Limit exposure to outdoor pollutants like traffic fumes and industrial emissions, especially during high pollution days.
    - Use air purifiers in your home,particularly in bedrooms.

- **Maintain good indoor air quality:**
    - Ensure proper ventilation in your home to remove indoor pollutants like dust, mold, and VOCs (volatile organic compounds) from furniture and cleaning products.
    - Regularly clean and dust surfaces,replace air filters, and address any dampness or mold issues promptly.

-

Allergens and Irritants:

- Identify and avoid personal triggers:
    - Common triggers include dust mites,pollen, mold, pet dander, and strong odors.
    - Keep pets out of bedrooms and wash bedding frequently.
    - Use hypoallergenic bedding and dust covers.

- Consider allergy testing to identify specific triggers and implement targeted avoidance strategies.
-
- **Control humidity levels:**
  - Maintain indoor humidity levels between 30-50% to prevent mold growth and dust mite proliferation.
  - Use a dehumidifier in damp climates.
-

Occupational Exposures:

- **Be aware of occupational hazards:**
  - Certain occupations expose individuals to dust, chemicals, or fumes that can irritate airways and exacerbate bronchiectasis symptoms.
  - Use appropriate personal protective equipment (PPE) like masks and gloves, as

recommended by your workplace safety policies.
  - Consider discussing alternative work arrangements with your employer if your current environment significantly aggravates your symptoms.
-

Lifestyle Practices:

- **Prioritize good hygiene:**
  - Frequent handwashing, especially after contact with potentially contaminated surfaces, helps prevent the spread of bacteria and viruses that can trigger lung infections.
  - Practice good dental hygiene to minimize upper respiratory tract infections.
-

- **Maintain a healthy lifestyle:**

- Eating a balanced diet rich in fruits,vegetables, and whole grains strengthens the immune system.
  - Regular exercise improves lung function and overall health.
  - Adequate sleep promotes immune function and recovery.
-

Additional Tips:

- **Travel with caution:**
  - Be mindful of air quality and potential allergen exposures while traveling,especially in areas with high pollution levels or unfamiliar climates.
  - Discuss preventive measures with your doctor before traveling, and carry necessary medications with you.
-
- **Manage stress:**

- Chronic stress can weaken the immune system and exacerbate symptoms.
- Practice stress management techniques like yoga, meditation, or deep breathing exercises.

Which foods are best to avoid if you have bronchiectasis

While there's no specific "forbidden food list" for bronchiectasis, certain dietary choices can contribute to lung irritation and exacerbate symptoms. By avoiding potential triggers and focusing on a balanced, lung-friendly diet, you can significantly improve your well-being and manage bronchiectasis effectively. Here's a breakdown of foods to minimize in your diet:

Foods high in inflammatory agents:

Processed meats: Hot dogs, sausages, deli meats, and bacon often contain preservatives and nitrates, which can trigger inflammation in the airways.

Sugary foods and drinks: High sugar intake promotes inflammation and can weaken the immune system, making you more susceptible to infections.

Fried foods: Deep-fried foods are high in saturated and trans fats, which can trigger inflammation and irritate the airways.

Dairy products: While research on dairy's impact on bronchiectasis is inconclusive, some individuals find that it thickens mucus and worsens symptoms. You can experiment with alternative milk options if you suspect dairy sensitivity.

Foods that may worsen mucus production:

Refined carbohydrates: White bread, pastries, and sugary cereals increase blood sugar levels, which can stimulate mucus production in some individuals. Opt for whole grains and complex carbohydrates instead.

Cow's milk: For some individuals, cow's milk can increase mucus production. Alternative milk options like oat milk or almond milk might be better tolerated.

Cruciferous vegetables: While generally healthy, cruciferous vegetables like broccoli, Brussels sprouts, and cabbage can sometimes cause bloating and gas, impacting breathing comfort. Moderation is key, and if they trigger discomfort, consider alternative vegetables.

Other potentially bothersome foods:

Spicy foods: For some individuals, spicy foods can irritate the airways and trigger coughing. Start with small amounts and observe your body's response.
Acidic foods: Tomatoes, citrus fruits, and vinegar can sometimes irritate the airways, especially for patients with gastroesophageal reflux disease (GERD). Experiment and identify what works best for you.

General Preventive Measures:

Healthy and balanced diet: Focus on fruits, vegetables, whole grains, lean protein, and healthy fats. These provide essential nutrients and antioxidants that support lung health.
Hydration: Drink plenty of water throughout the day to thin mucus and keep airways hydrated.
Regular exercise: Maintain physical activity to strengthen your respiratory system and improve overall health.

Smoking cessation: Smoking is a major trigger for bronchiectasis and worsens symptoms significantly. Quitting smoking is crucial for managing the condition.

Manage other health conditions: Address any underlying conditions like allergies, sinus infections, or GERD, as they can contribute to bronchiectasis symptoms.

Regular consultations: Maintain regular appointments with your doctor to monitor your condition and adjust treatment plans as needed.

NOTE: Every individual with bronchiectasis is different, and food triggers can vary. Pay attention to how your body reacts to different foods and adjust your diet accordingly.

CHAPTER SEVEN

Natural and Herbal Approaches

While conventional treatment remains essential for managing bronchiectasis, some natural and herbal approaches can complement therapy and promote overall well-being. It's important to remember that these approaches are not replacements for conventional treatment and should always be discussed with your doctor before initiation.

Exploring Natural Remedies

Natural Approaches:

Steam therapy: Inhaling warm, moist air helps loosen mucus and ease congestion. Use a humidifier or take hot showers with closed doors.

Chest percussion: Gentle tapping on the chest can help dislodge mucus. Ask your doctor or physiotherapist for proper technique.

Postural drainage: Lying in specific positions with head lowered can assist in draining mucus from different lung segments. Learn the postures from a healthcare professional.

Hydration: Drinking plenty of water and fluids keeps mucus thin and easier to clear. Aim for 8-10 glasses per day.

Saltwater gargle: Gargling with warm saltwater can soothe a sore throat and reduce inflammation. Use half a teaspoon of salt in a glass of warm water.

Herbal Approaches:

Ginger: has anti-inflammatory and antioxidant properties that can help reduce inflammation of the respiratory tract and improve lung function. You can use ginger in the form of tea, add it to food or take it as additives.

Turmeric: Curcumin, the active component of turmeric, has anti-inflammatory and antibacterial properties that can help reduce inflammation of the respiratory tract and fight infections. You can use turmeric as a spice, add it to food or take it as additives.

N-acetylcysteine (NAC): NAC is an antioxidant that helps to thin mucus and facilitate its removal from the lungs. NAC can be taken as supplements.

Echinacea: Echinacea is considered an immunostimulatory that can help strengthen the immune system and fight infections. However, keep in mind that studies on the effectiveness of echinacea in bronchiectasis are limited.

Oregano: Oregano can help relieve the symptoms of cough and bronchitis. It can be consumed in the form of tea or inhalation.

Important Points:

Safety first: Ensure the herbs you choose are safe for you and don't interact with any medications you're taking.

Quality matters: Choose high-quality herbs from reputable sources.

Start slow: Begin with small doses and gradually increase if tolerated.

Monitor closely: Pay attention to how your body reacts and discontinue use if you experience any adverse effects.

Consult your doctor: Always inform your doctor about any herbal remedies you're considering or using.

Herbal Therapies

Potential Benefits of Herbal Therapies in Bronchiectasis:

Anti-inflammatory properties: Certain herbs like turmeric, ginger, and licorice root may possess anti-inflammatory properties that could potentially reduce airway inflammation and irritation.
Mucus clearing and expectorant effects: Herbs like marshmallow root, mullein, and elderberry may help loosen mucus and promote expectoration, easing breathing and reducing cough.

Antimicrobial effects: Some herbs like garlic, oregano, and echinacea are known for their antimicrobial properties, potentially aiding in fighting off infections that can exacerbate bronchiectasis.

Immune system support: Herbs like astragalus and ginseng may offer some immune system support, potentially helping the body fight off infections and manage the condition.

Important Cautions and Considerations:

Limited research: Most herbal remedies lack strong scientific evidence supporting their effectiveness in bronchiectasis. Their benefits are often anecdotal and require further research.

Potential interactions: Herbs can interact with conventional medications, potentially causing adverse effects. Consult your doctor before using any herbal remedies to avoid harmful interactions.

Dosage and quality: Proper dosage and quality control are crucial with herbal remedies. Consult a qualified herbalist or healthcare professional for guidance on safe and effective usage.

Potential side effects: Herbs can have side effects, and individuals with certain health conditions may not tolerate them well.

Be aware of potential side effects and consult your doctor before using any herbal remedies.

Not a substitute for conventional treatment:
Herbal remedies should not replace conventional
bronchiectasis treatment. They should be used as
complementary therapies alongside prescribed
medications as advised by your doctor.

Examples of Potentially Helpful Herbs:

Turmeric: Anti-inflammatory properties may help
reduce airway inflammation.
Ginger: Anti-inflammatory and expectorant
properties may ease cough and loosen mucus.
Marshmallow root: Soothing and expectorant
properties may help soothe irritated airways and
loosen mucus.
Mullein: Traditionally used for respiratory issues,
may help loosen mucus and ease cough.
Elderberry: May offer some immune support and
antiviral properties.

"Breathing Freely, Living Fully"

As we reach the closing chapter of "Overcoming Bronchiectasis: A Step-by-Step Guide," the journey we've embarked on together reveals the resilience of the human spirit and the power of knowledge, community, and perseverance in the face of bronchiectasis.

For patients like Helen, the pages of this guide represent not just medical advice but a roadmap to reclaiming life. It's a testament to the progress that can be made when individuals, armed with understanding and supported by dedicated healthcare providers, approach bronchiectasis as a challenge to be faced head-on.

To health care providers, this guide stands as a collaborative tool, offering insights into the multifaceted care required for bronchiectasis patients. By combining medical expertise with empathy, you play a pivotal role in transforming lives and fostering hope.

As we conclude this journey, let it be a reminder that overcoming bronchiectasis is not a solitary pursuit. It is a collective effort, with patients, healthcare providers, and communities working hand in hand. Breathing freely is not just a physical act but a metaphor for living fully, embracing every moment with gratitude and determination.

May this guide serve as a source of empowerment, a beacon of hope, and a reminder that, together, we can triumph over the challenges of bronchiectasis. Let each page echo the resilience of those who face this condition, and may the stories within inspire a future where every breath is a celebration of life.

As we bid farewell to these pages, let it be with the understanding that the journey continues. New chapters await, filled with possibilities, progress, and the unwavering spirit of those who refuse to be defined by bronchiectasis. Here's to breathing freely and living fully.